The
POWER
of
Ancient
Wellness

First published in Great Britain in 2023 by
Michael O'Mara Books Limited
9 Lion Yard
Tremadoc Road
London SW4 7NQ

This product is made of material from well-managed, FSC®-certified forests and other controlled sources. The manufacturing processes conform to the environmental regulations of the country of origin.

ISBN: 978-1-78929-597-9 in paperback print format
ISBN: 978-1-78929-600-6 in ebook format

1 2 3 4 5 6 7 8 9 10

This book contains advice including instructions and recipes for remedies that are FOR GUIDANCE ONLY and should not be relied upon as an alternative to professional advice from either your doctor or a registered specialist. You are strongly recommended to consult a doctor if you have any medical or other physical concerns. Neither the publisher nor the author can accept any responsibility for any consequences that may follow if such specialist advice is not sought.

Cover design by Natasha Le Coultre
using illustrations by Anna Stead, licensed by Jehane Ltd.
Designed by Natasha Le Coultre and Barbara Ward
Illustrations © Anna Stead Licensed by Jehane Ltd.

Printed and bound in China

www.mombooks.com

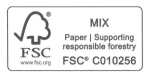

MIX
Paper | Supporting
responsible forestry
FSC® C010256

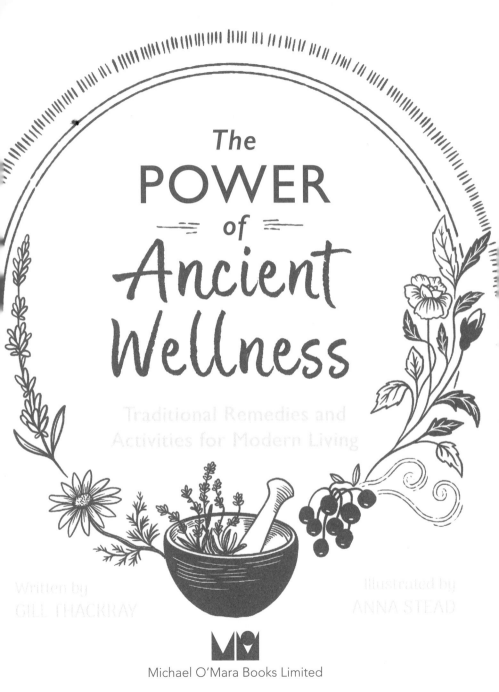

The
POWER
of
Ancient
Wellness

Traditional Remedies and
Activities for Modern Living

Written by
GILL THACKRAY

Illustrated by
ANNA STEAD

Michael O'Mara Books Limited

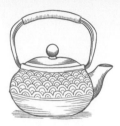

Contents

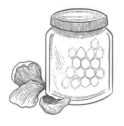

BODY

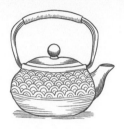

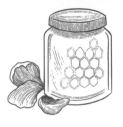

A Healing Massage with Gua Sha
97

Inner and Outer Beauty with Plant-based Masks
100

SPIRIT

Restore Equilibrium with Limpia
109

Open Your Heart with a Cacao Ceremony
112

The Healing Power of Trees
116

Healing and Cleansing Waters
121

Nature Is Therapy, Wherever You Are
124

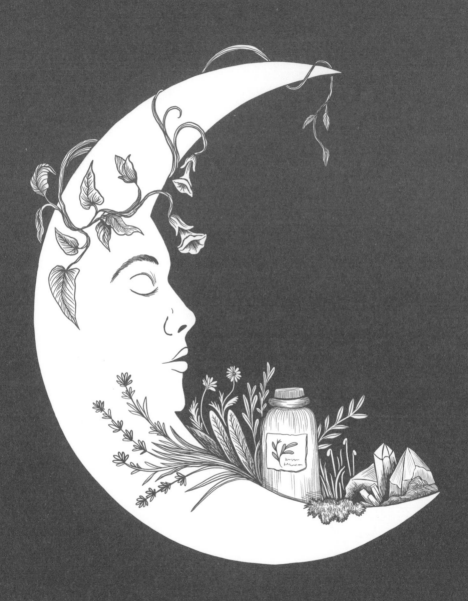

Introduction

The ancient world moved to a different rhythm. Our ancestors' lives were slower. They lived in tune with natural cycles that we in modern society have become disconnected from. We move at such speed that anxiety, stress, workplace burnout and insomnia are endemic. Even as we sleep, our brains are milling and grinding, hard at work attempting to process the overwhelm. Our bodies and minds are set to an unsustainable survival mode, and we feel it.

A new movement is emerging to live more deliberately, embracing the old ways and recognizing that we're a fundamental part of the natural world. We're not separate from it and never have been. This is the indigenous knowledge of our ancestors. Somewhere deep inside us, if we become still enough, we can hear it. By listening to that wisdom, we can meet our true selves, build our resilience, raise our consciousness and move through the world with unshakeable calm.

In *The Power of Ancient Wellness*, you'll discover some of the oldest healing techniques in existence, to create serenity, improve sleep and boost your wellbeing. You'll find breathwork techniques to put the brakes on stress and botanical rituals to reconnect with the wild, natural world that each of us belongs to. We'll also examine how exciting new scientific research corroborates what our ancestors knew intuitively. This book is divided into three pathways:

Mind

Body   Spirit

In each section, you'll journey through a series of powerful ancient wellness practices for a modern world. You'll learn to create your own customized, holistic toolkit with simple, intuitive daily rituals and to connect with the botany of your local landscape to improve your wellbeing though traditional tinctures, healing balms and more. These ancient teachings will help you to align with your true purpose and optimize your health.

You'll discover potent energy medicine practices to awaken your spirituality along with transformational nature-based therapies and rituals to decompress your mind, body and soul. This timeless, ancient wisdom will teach you wellness principles to reconnect with your own innate capacity for inner healing, peace and joy. Listen to the ancients calling you to pause and realign. As the first-century sage Hillel enquired, if not now, then when?

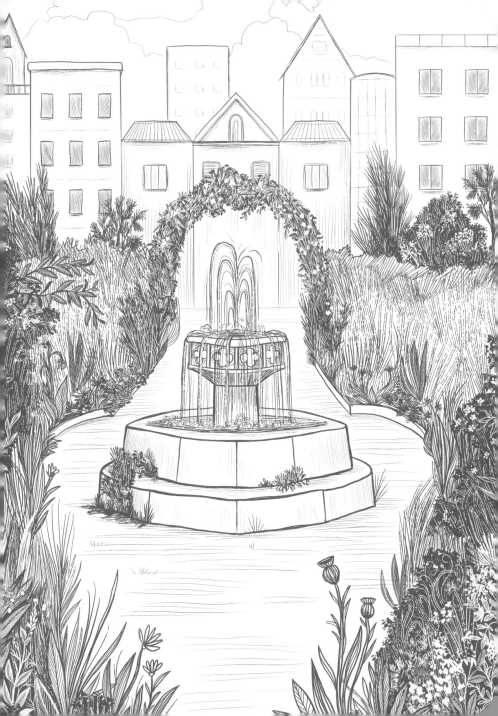

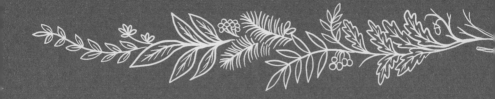

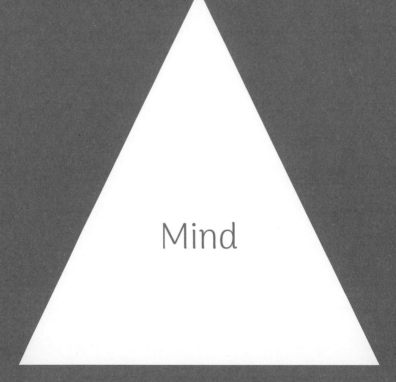

Mind

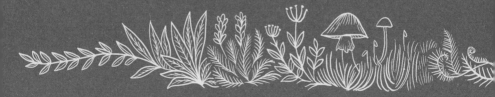

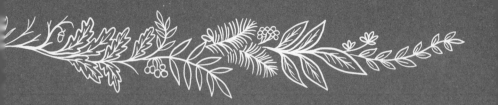

The frenetic pace of life can often leave us feeling unmoored and destabilized. Bringing awareness to each day, leaving autopilot behind by adopting a more mindful approach to daily life, can be transformational. In this section you'll discover how to live more consciously with ancient practices that are designed to help you slow down. Reconnect with the power of the divine feminine. Learn how nature can be a powerful antidote to modern stress. Explore how to shape your reality (along with your neural networks) by changing your mindset.

Engaging with the foundational tools in this section will help you to heal unresolved wounds and connect with your innate joy, compassion and boundless self-love. Fearlessly live your truth with these sustainable daily wellness practices.

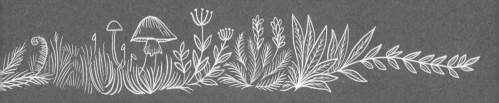

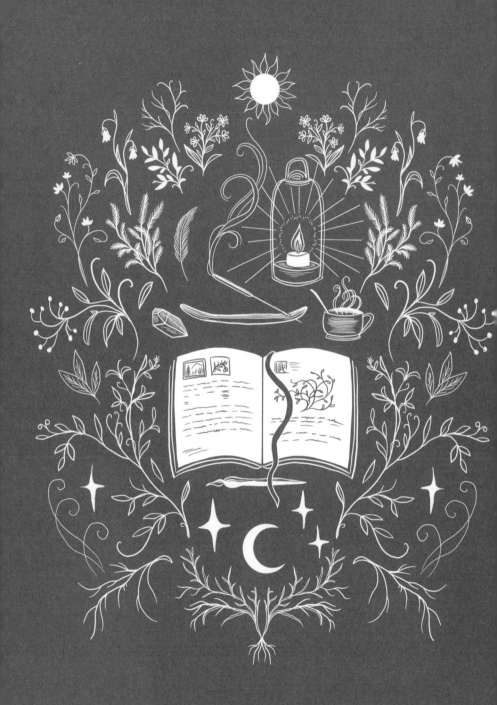

The Power of Rituals

Daily rituals and ceremonies are profound wellness practices that ground us, allowing us to touch base with ourselves and the universe. Harvard professor Mike Norton's research found that people who regularly used rituals felt positive, less overwhelmed and more in control of their lives. The energy we send out is the energy we get back.

Rituals are acts that we repeat over time. They are different to habits, as we do them with intention. Rituals energize and empower us, help us to focus and remind us of our innate wisdom. We can incorporate them into everything we do. Daily, weekly or monthly rituals can be acts of personal devotion, such as taking time to light a candle or burn incense, as well as journaling or offering thanks before a meal.

Exercise: Morning tea ritual

Consider applying ceremonial principles to simple daily activities, such as drinking tea. Meditative Japanese tea ceremonies, or *chanoyu* (茶の湯), date back to the ninth century, with roots in Zen Buddhism. When you're struggling to find your equilibrium, a five-minute tea ceremony provides a soothing way of turning inward and recentering yourself. Dial down the sensory overload with the preparation of tea and, if you're able to, enjoy your drink in nature to amplify the wellness benefits.

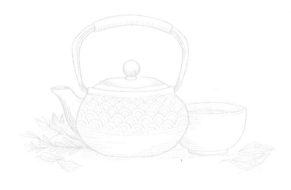

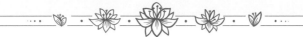

1. Choose a reusable cup that appeals to you. Pause and reflect.

2. Bring meaning to the preparation of your tea. Soak in each moment, from boiling the water to inhaling the aroma emanating from your cup.

3. Focus on where you are in the day. Notice the ebb and flow of life around you. Notice how you feel.

4. Set an intention for the rest of your day. What would you like more of? Is there something that you would like to do less of? Or an area where you want to focus your attention?

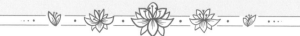

Exercise: Build a sacred sanctuary

A sanctuary can be a simple corner, a chair or an uncomplicated altar. If the beauty and wisdom of the natural world evokes peace for you, choose a spot on a balcony, in a garden or somewhere in the local landscape as your portal to peace. Your own zen-den for reflection, meditation, ritual and ceremony can be a powerful, deeply nourishing and supportive space. Think of it as a place for self-care, a harmonious refuge away from the daily grind.

If space is an issue, don't worry. Your sanctuary doesn't have to take up an entire room. You can even create a portable sanctuary by choosing a handful of small items, such as crystals or an image of a spiritual figure that inspires and connects you to the divine. Traditionally, the energy of a space is cleansed and purified by drumming or using bells.

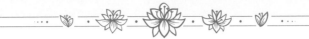

Before you begin, ask yourself:

What is your intention for this space?

How will you use this sanctuary?

What will you need to create balance and
harmony? Meditation cushions, aromatherapy
oils, books, candles, crystals, creative supplies?
A cluttered sanctuary can add to internal stress,
so keep it simple.

How can you interweave your sanctuary into
your daily routine?

Connect with the Divine Feminine

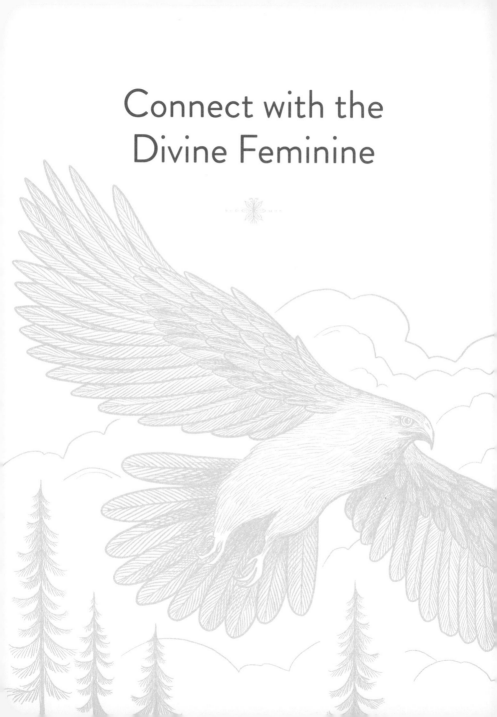

The divine feminine and divine masculine are sacred energies that exist in *all* living things. It's the yin and yang of the universe. We hold both forces within us, irrespective of how we identify. Ancient civilizations revered and worshipped the divine feminine as an equal counterpart to the divine masculine. Both masculine and feminine energies were balanced – until something changed. We began to rely solely on the masculine and the feminine was diminished, demoted and devalued.

Indigenous traditions have compared humanity to a bird flying with only the masculine wing. This has created imbalance in the world. We're out of alignment, flying around in a circle. Cherokee prophecy holds that the twenty-first century will see the feminine wing fully extend and balance will be restored. Only then will the bird of humanity soar.

For decades, there has been a re-emergence of the divine feminine. A recognition that we need to reconnect to the archetype of that powerful, healing feminine found in so many indigenous cultures. When we're balanced within, we can send that energy out into the world.

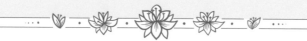

Exercise: Goddess meditation

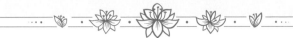

1. Get into a comfortable seated position with your feet flat on the floor. Relax and soften your body.

2. Breathe in through your nose and out through your mouth. Focus on your breath, settling into a gentle rhythm.

3. Notice your feet connecting with the ground. As you absorb that energy from the earth, connect with the divine feminine within you. Visualize a warm, nurturing light glowing in your heart centre. Bathe in this restorative, healing energy. Feel her power, her strength and her courage.

4. Feel the energy of this light vibrating throughout your entire body. Notice how it illuminates every cell. Now picture that energy emanating outwards into the universe. Rest in this healing space for five minutes.

Realign with Mother Earth with Moon Bathing

The mystical, fluid energy of the moon was honored by the Incas. Worshipping celestial bodies was central to this ancient culture. The moon, or Mama Killa (pronounced *Kee-yah*) as she is known, is the heavenly grandmother, watching over the earth. There are four major lunar phases: new moon, first quarter, full moon and last quarter. Each phase lasts approximately seven and a half days, with a full cycle of the moon, or *lunation*, taking twenty-nine and a half days.

Around the world, across cultures, the waxing and waning of Grandmother Moon has informed calendars, time, planting, harvests, travel and tradition for generations. Each moon cycle has its own unique, sacred energy.

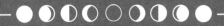

New moon
Set your intentions. Decide what you want
to call in for yourself, your community
and the world.

✦

First quarter
Take time for self-compassion and self-care
and act on your goals.

✦

Full moon
Reflect on where you are and manifest
what you've yet to achieve.

✦

Last quarter
Find gratitude for what you've received from
the universe. Let go of what you no longer
need before the cycle begins again with
the next new moon.

Exercise: Moon bathing

The ancient wisdom of the Incas incorporates moon bathing as a way of releasing heavy energy. Work with the lunar phases to strengthen self-care, set intentions, let go of what you no longer need and connect with the divine energy of the universe. Reaching out to this mystical lunar energy is a great way to connect with the natural world. Think of this as a time to reflect on where you are and where you'd like to be spiritually, emotionally and physically.

1. Bring a calm, open mind and spirit of gratitude to your moon bathing.

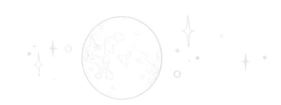

2. Spend time grounding. If your mind is leaping from one thought to another, consciously turn inwards and meditate for a few minutes to settle your internal energies.

3. Set an intention for your moon bath. This could be something that you're grateful for and would like to celebrate and give thanks for, a part of your life that you'd like to release and let go of, or an energy or situation that you would like to manifest into the world.

4. Find a comfortable spot (indoors or outdoors) in moonlight. Feel the healing light of the moon fall upon you.

5. Spend as much time as you need bathing in the moonlight and visualize your intention.

6. When you've finished, express gratitude to Grandmother Moon.

Connect with Nature Barefoot

Known as earthing (and grounding), walking barefoot and connecting with the earth feels sublime. Whether it's sinking your toes into powder-soft, warm sand or the vibrant, revitalizing sensation of soft, wet grass underfoot at the beginning of a summer's day, connecting with nature restores

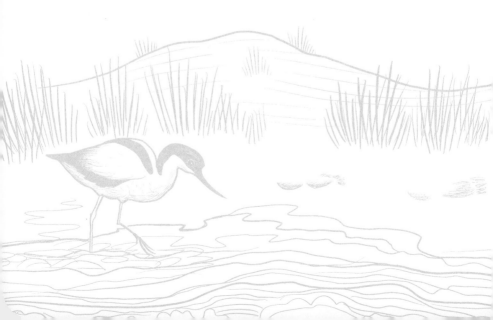

and rejuvenates our mind and body. What's more, studies have found that barefoot earthing produces measurable differences in the concentrations of white blood cells and cytokines, improving our immune response.

Our ancestors walked barefoot, directly connecting with the earth's energies. Indigenous cultures around the world acknowledged the powerful, therapeutic power of the earth. In traditional Chinese medicine, this energy is referred to as *'earth qi'*. Sioux Native Americans recognized the power of connecting with the earth centuries before studies analyzing the healing properties of soil. Simply going shoeless for thirty minutes can improve our wellness on multiple levels.

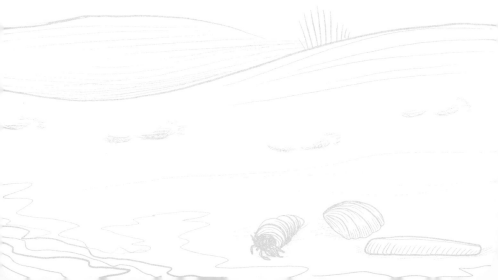

Exercise: Barefoot earthing exercise

1. Find a natural outdoor space clear of stones and debris.

2. Kick your shoes and socks off and make direct barefoot contact with the earth.

3. See if it's possible to make earthing a regular practice, integrating it into your daily rituals.

4. Reflect on how you feel after your earthing session.

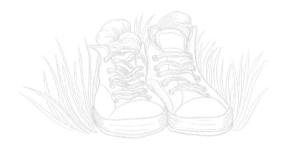

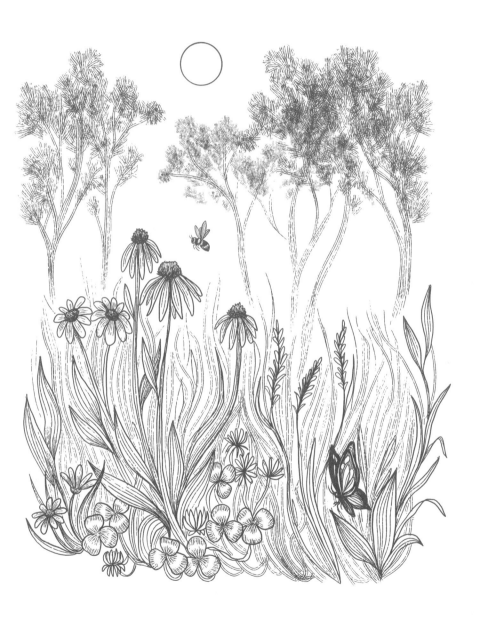

Embrace a Toltec Mindset

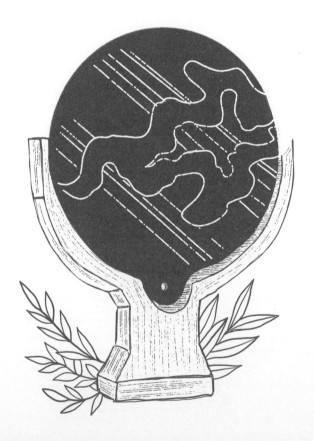

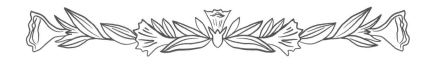

Inner knowing – we all have it, even if, in a world full of noise, tuning into this source of power can feel like unchartered territory. But when we're able to dial down our mental chatter, our innate wisdom is there, waiting for us. This philosophy is grounded in the powerful wisdom of the Toltec civilization from tenth-century Mexico.

The Toltecs believed that mindset was crucial. They recognized that our world is like a mirror obscured by smoke. The habitual thought patterns, inner critic, imposter syndrome and limiting beliefs we learn become a barrier to our innate wisdom.

Modern-day life moves too frantically to hear the whisper of this inner compass. We get lost in the foggy autopilot of our own smoky mirror. The Toltecs knew nothing of neuroscience, but we now understand from studies into mindset and neuroplasticity (the brain's ability to change) that we can rewire old habits and thought patterns. When we change the way we think, we can change our reality. Learn to trust your inner wisdom by following these simple steps.

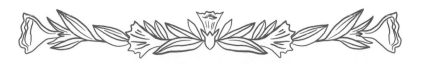

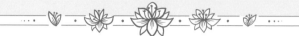

Exercise: Toltec mindset

1. Monitor and identify your thinking patterns. Begin to recognize the worn out, unhelpful thoughts that are keeping you stuck and stressed.

2. Examine your stories. Where have you created stories that are keeping you stuck? Which stories are part of your becoming, moving you forwards?

3. When you're faced with a question, meditate and ground yourself. Embrace the sacredness of becoming still.

4. Ask yourself: what is the answer for my highest good? How can I evolve my consciousness? What will move me towards my potential?

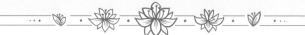

5. Write down your question. Allow your inner voice to respond with an answer. Listen and connect to the guidance that appears on each page.

6. It may be a quiet voice at first, but the more you connect with it, the louder and clearer your inner wisdom will become.

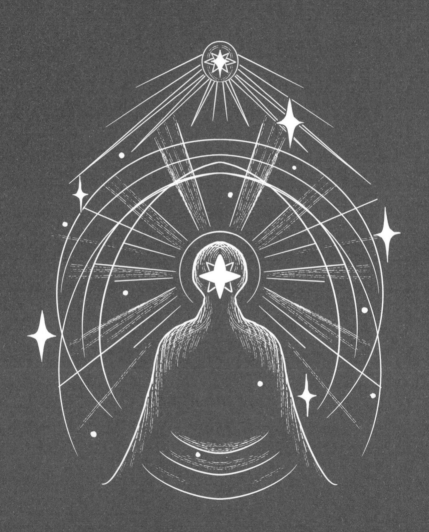

The Power of Protection with Wiracocha

The wisdom of the Peruvian Qero is recognized around the globe. Sometimes referred to as the last of the Incas, they worship Mother Earth (*Pachamama* in the Quechua language). The Qero believe that through living in balance, practising *ayni* (reciprocity) with the earth, we can heal ourselves, each other and the world.

The Qero have a special practice for protecting their energy, known as the 'opening of wiracocha'. This is the halo of light found directly above the crown of the head, sometimes referred to as our soul star or spirit bubble. Believed to be the connection between your physical and spiritual body, it links us to the universe. According to the Qero, by opening wiracocha, our life force energy, we're able to expand that sacred, protective light around ourselves.

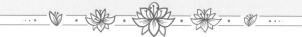

Exercise: Opening of wiracocha

By reaching into the sacred space directly above the crown of your head, you can access and wrap your wiracocha around your physical body to create a sacred space, protect yourself and connect with the universal energy that surrounds all of us.

1. Bring your hands together in prayer pose in front of your heart.

2. With intention, reach upwards with your arms and hands over your head, maintaining prayer pose. When your hands are directly above your crown, reverse your palms.

3. Draw the sacred energy of your wiracocha all around your body, sweeping your hands and arms along your sides and down to the earth.

4. Use your fingertips to direct any remaining energy towards Pachamama in thanks.

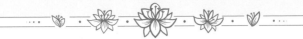

5. Notice how it feels as you bathe in the light of your wiracocha.

6. When you have completion or no longer need to keep your wiracocha open, close it by placing open palms toward the earth by your sides.

7. Sweep your arms upwards, gathering the hem of your energy field all the way up back towards your eighth chakra.

8. Once your hands reach above your crown, pause. With palms facing towards your body, draw some of this golden energy down into each chakra.

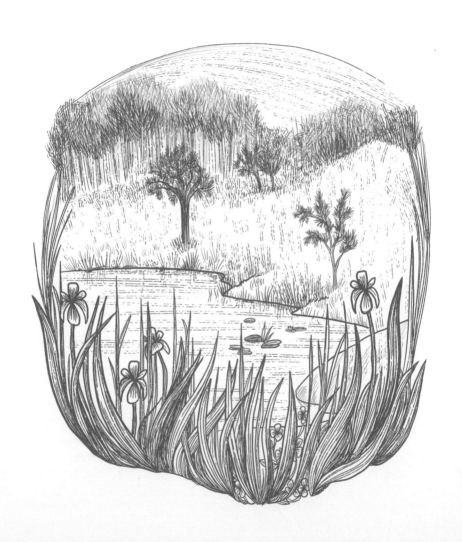

Find Calm with Ancient Mindful Decoupling

When you're in the grip of anxiety – whether caused by workload, a disagreement or an upcoming event weighing on your mind – it's easy to feel triggered. Fear, overwhelm and anxiety is our autonomic nervous system placing us on high alert. It's our fight, flight, freeze response activated by a part of our brain called the amygdala. That response can easily push us into overload, dysregulating our emotions and making it difficult to think with clarity.

Mindfulness has been used for centuries to help reduce pain, fear and anxiety. The process of decoupling helps us to see that our thoughts are not necessarily facts. Sometimes thoughts are just mental events. Mindful decoupling activates our parasympathetic nervous system, allowing us to slow down and come back to our natural state of calm.

Exercise: Mindfulness

The next time you feel triggered by an uncomfortable thought or find yourself in the grip of incessant negativity, try this powerful reflection.

1. Become present in the moment. Set an intention to decouple from the stress trigger.

2. Follow the breath all the way in and all the way out. As you focus on each breath, you're bringing your nervous system into balance. Do this for a few minutes, or as long as you feel is necessary.

3. As thoughts arise, notice if you automatically jump to a conclusion. Ask yourself, is it true? How does this thought leave me feeling? What would I feel like if I didn't believe this?

4. When you begin to feel centred, continue to breathe slowly and steadily for a few more moments before bringing the meditation to an end.

Restore Balance
with a Gratitude Ritual

The practice of gratitude has an impressive body of research behind it. Studies into positive psychology at the University of Pennsylvania found that regularly experiencing gratitude increased happiness by 25 per cent. What's more, keeping a gratitude journal improved sleep quantity and quality. There is a wellspring of mind–body benefits associated with gratitude, from heart health, optimism and feeling less stressed, to increased levels of the happiness hormone oxytocin and longevity. But this isn't a new concept.

Giving thanks has been seen as crucial for physical and spiritual health for centuries. The Greco-Roman world considered it a prerequisite for a life well lived. Buddhism even has practices to mindfully send gratitude to your enemies.

A profound wellness practice, gratitude helps us to reimagine our lives from a place of abundance rather than what we don't have. So it's not difficult to see how, throughout history, gratitude has been used to restore inner and outer balance.

Consciously set aside time at the end of each day to build a ritual of thankfulness. By making this an evening practice, you'll be able to train yourself to look for opportunities to be grateful throughout the day. That means that you'll be amplifying the benefits through self-directed neuroplasticity, hardwiring your brain for happiness.

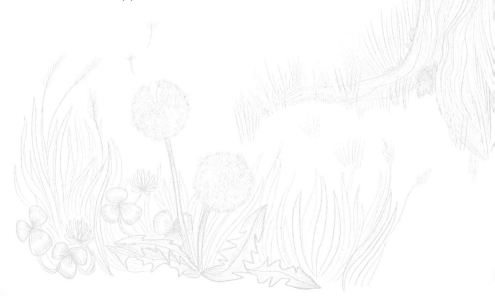

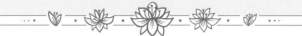

Exercise: Gratitude

Decide on a time for your gratitude ritual. If you link it to an existing habit – for example, a bedtime routine – you'll increase the chance of maintaining it. You'll need a pen and paper, or, better still, a journal by your bedside.

1. Reflect on your day. Write down three things that you're grateful for. It could be something simple like the sun shining, a lesson that the day taught you or time spent engaged in an activity you love.

2. Make each sentence as detailed as you can. Write down what happened and how it made you feel.

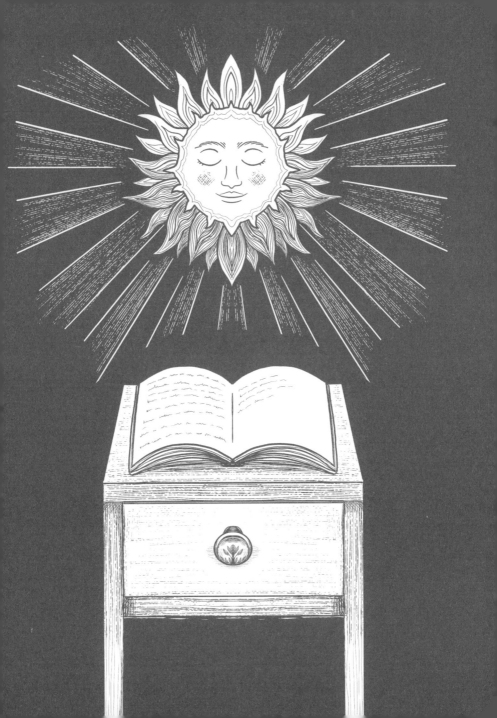

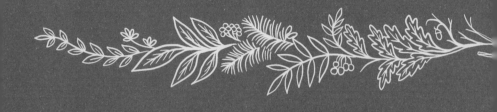

Body

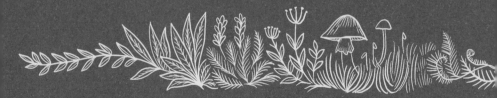

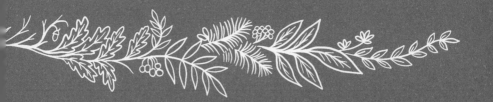

Harness centuries-old wellness traditions to bring your body back into balance. In this section you'll explore how to repair, restore and optimize your physical health with the old ways. Create an ancient apothecary with botanicals used to treat physical and mental disease for centuries. Develop bespoke medicinal preparations to aid sleep, elicit calm and foster intense focus. Draw upon biodynamic ancient foods to supercharge your vitality. Learn how to clear stagnant energy in the subtle realms beyond the physical world and manage stress with self-reiki.

These techniques have endured for thousands of years. The wisdom in this section will help you to self-regulate physically and emotionally, ushering in a healthier, more authentic and fulfilling life, inside and out.

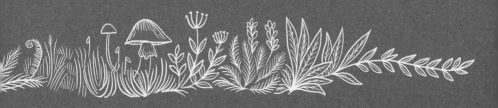

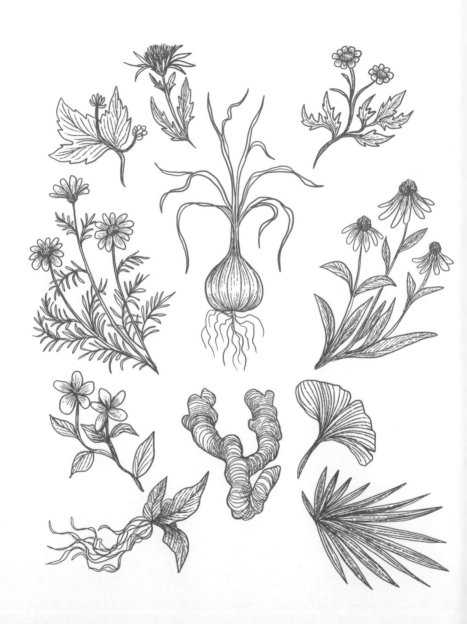

Your Ancient Apothecary

Plants have a natural intelligence – we just need to tune into it. Working with botanicals to create your own ancient apothecary provides an opportunity to transcend the busyness of everyday life. Familiarize yourself with native plants and herbs in your area, getting to know their physical and energetic properties. You'll discover that seemingly simple botanical ingredients have a powerful effect on your health and your spirit. Invite in an even deeper connection with the natural world by growing your own herbs.

Tinctures are potent plant infusions used to extract and preserve active botanical properties. Herbs used in tinctures are chosen for their healing properties. Once you've mastered the elements that comprise a basic tincture, you can begin to explore your favourite medicinal plants and herbs to create your own natural pharmacy.

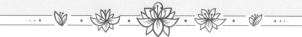

Exercise: Basic tincture method

1. Collect enough of your chosen medicinal herbs to fill a jar. Roughly crush or chop, then add the plant to a sterilized container. Where you can, use fresh leaves and herbs for potency. If that's not possible, you can use dried ingredients instead.

2. Fill your jar with undiluted apple cider vinegar, which has the additional benefit of probiotics to support your gut microbiome.

3. Allow the tincture to infuse in a cool, dark place, gently releasing the botanical compounds, for four weeks or longer. Shake the jar daily to aid the process.

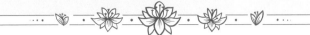

4. After the tincture has infused, filter through a muslin cloth and funnel. Discard the herbs (they're compostable).

5. Decant into a sterile dropper bottle and label. It will last for eight to twelve months.

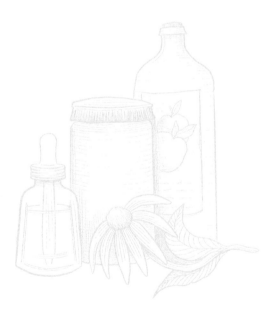

⊸ ∘ ∘ Sleep: ∘ ∘ ⊶
Lemon balm tincture

Known for its medicinal properties, lemon balm (*Melissa officinalis*) promotes sleep, alleviates anxiety and reduces stress, creating the foundation for a restful, rejuvenating night. You will need two cups of lemon balm leaves for this tincture. Place three drops on your tongue before bedtime.

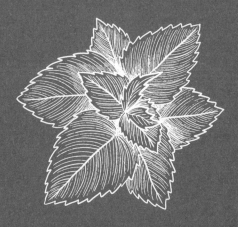

⊸ ∘ ∘ Stress and anxiety: ∘ ∘ ⊱
Lavender and chamomile tincture

Associated with calm and elevated mood for centuries, lavender (*Lavandula*) has a natural affinity with anxiety reduction. The phytochemicals in chamomile (*Matricaria recutita*) also possess emotionally soothing properties. Use half a cup of lavender flowers and half a cup of chamomile flowers to make your tincture. Place a few drops on your tongue and temples when you need to find a moment of calm.

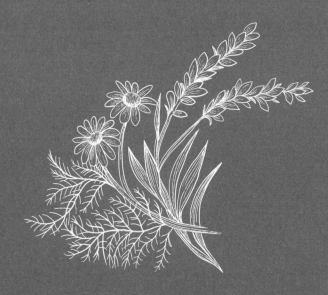

⊸∘∘ Focus: ∘∘⊶
Rosemary tincture

Rosemary (*Salvia rosmarinus*) has been used in folk medicine for hundreds of years. Researchers at Northumbria University found that active compounds in rosemary have a positive effect on learning and memory, improving performance. You will need two cups of fresh rosemary or one cup if it is dried. Use this powerful tincture whenever you need clarity at work, to focus while studying or you just want to be at the top of your game.

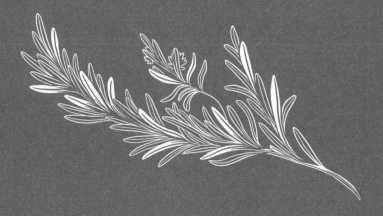

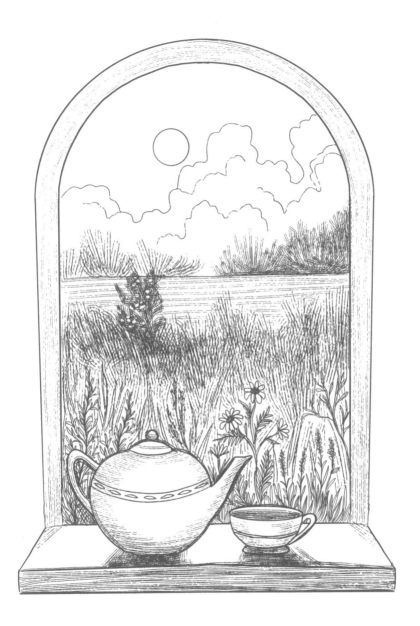

Your Ancient Superfood Staples

Our gut is sometimes referred to as our second brain. Diet and digestion impact our mental and physical health, playing a crucial role in fighting some diseases. What we put into our body shapes our mood, affecting all the bodily systems. The tradition of phytomedicine, using some of the same roots, berries, plants and seeds as our ancestors, has long been a wellness staple, helping to strengthen our immune system. Here are some of the most powerful ancient superfoods on the planet.

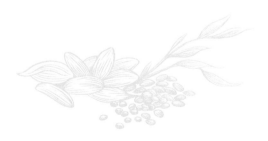

Oats

One of the oldest grains on earth, oats (*Avena sativa*) were used by ancient cultures in a variety of ways. Archaeological evidence suggests that Palaeolithic societies ground them into flour. Early Egyptians used them as cosmetics; the Celts cultivated them for food and our Bronze Age ancestors fed oats to their cattle. Today, the humble oat has many wellness benefits. The anti-inflammatory compounds improve our gut microbiome and may help with the prevention of some diseases.

You can add a tablespoon to smoothies, sprinkled on yoghurt or – a traditional favourite – eat in the form of porridge. Overnight oats are simply oats that have been mixed with milk, plant milk or water and left to soak overnight. If you can, use steel-cut oats, as they are minimally processed, contain the highest amount of fibre and have a lower glycaemic index, making them better for blood sugar control.

Flax

One of the oldest crops on the planet, flax or linseed is the ultimate superfood. In ancient Egypt, blue flowered flax was considered a symbol of purity. Neolithic and Viking cultures used the fibre from this incredible plant to create textiles (linen), rope, baskets, paper, oil and fishing nets. Today, flaxseed is a wellness plant ally.

The powerful active components of flaxseed are used to help reduce cholesterol, manage diabetes, alleviate menopausal symptoms and maintain gut health. What's more, flax is packed with lignans – phytochemicals that research suggests may protect against certain types of cancer. Use ground flax to maximize its wellness properties. You can add one to two tablespoons daily to smoothies, yoghurt, cereals, porridge or as a salad topping. If you're vegan, flax makes an excellent egg substitute, mixed with water and known as a 'flax egg'.

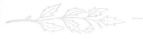

Chia

Chia (*Salvia columbariae*) was used by pre-Columbian civilizations for food, pressed for oil, used medicinally and added to drinks. The Mayans offered chia ceremonially to Aztec gods, believing that it manifested supernatural powers of strength and stamina. Loaded with healthy omega-3 fatty acids along with anti-inflammatory quercetin, chia seeds have been linked to the prevention of high blood pressure, strokes and heart disease.

Chia seeds can be added to baking, cereal, smoothies and granola. One of the easiest ways of eating this super-healthy grain is in a delicious chia pudding. Simply mix half a cup of chia seeds with one cup of milk of your choice. Give it a good stir to separate the seeds. Add a handful of blueberries, cardamom, maple syrup or date paste to taste, and leave to set in the refrigerator.

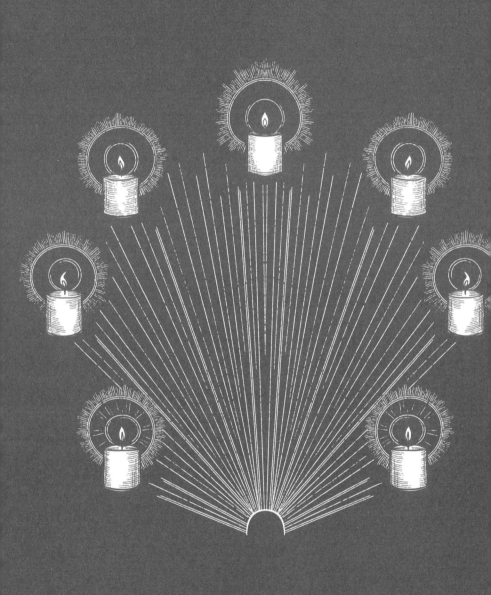

Remove Energetic Blocks with Chakra-clearing

Meaning 'wheel' in Sanskrit, the ancient energy system 'chakra' can be traced all the way back to the sacred Vedas text. Found in Hindu and Buddhist traditions, along with Kundalini and Ayurveda practices, chakras are believed to be energy centres responsible for the flow of energy. They are where your physical and energetic body intersect. We can't see them, and although there's no way of empirically measuring the chakras, you may sense them with practice. Running all the way from the base of the spine to the crown of the head, these vortices maintain the energetic balance in the body. Over time, Ayurvedic, Hindu and Buddhist belief systems have all taken a different approach to the chakra system. Typically, the main energy points can be viewed as eight major chakras, each governing a different area of your life.

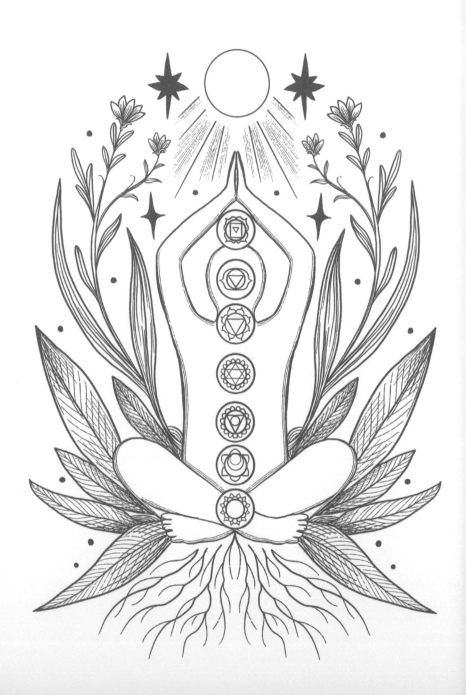

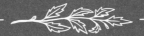

 8. Soul chakra (Murdhanta). White. Your spiritual connection to the universe.

 7. Crown chakra (Sahasrara). White or violet. Representing spirituality and purpose.

 6. Third-eye chakra (Ajna). Indigo. Intuition and instinct.

 5. Throat chakra (Visuddha). Blue. Where your internal world meets the outer world to speak your truth.

 4. Heart chakra (Anahata). Green. Love, compassion, forgiveness and intimacy.

 3. Solar plexus chakra (Manipura). Yellow. Responsible for confidence, self-esteem and safety.

 2. Sacral chakra (Svadhisthana). Orange. The seat of creativity and emotions.

 1. Root chakra (Muladhara). Red. Responsible for your sense of safety, trust and groundedness.

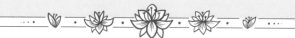

Exercise: Chakra-clearing

When your chakras are running clean and clear, everything feels harmonious. When these energy centres are blocked, you'll feel out of balance physically, emotionally and spiritually. You may notice that you feel heightened stress, have trouble sleeping or perhaps you're quick to jump to conclusions. When you feel your energy is misaligned or stagnant, this nurturing practice will remove blocks, restoring balance to your energy pathways.

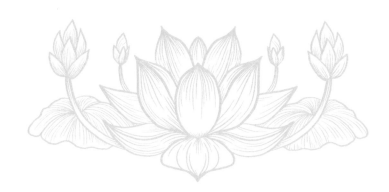

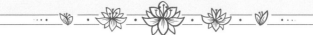

1. Create an intention to clear any blockages from your chakras.

2. Check in with each chakra. See if it's possible to decipher the subtle energy within your internal landscape.

3. Working from the crown of your head, use your hand to spin your chakra in a circular motion counter-clockwise, three times. This releases any stagnant or blocked energy. Repeat this unwinding gesture on each chakra, working all the way down to your root chakra. Visualize the stagnant energy draining into the earth.

4. Once you've unwound all eight chakras, return to the crown of the head. This time, spin each chakra clockwise to reset it. Visualize each chakra cleansed, restored and overflowing with a warm, healing light.

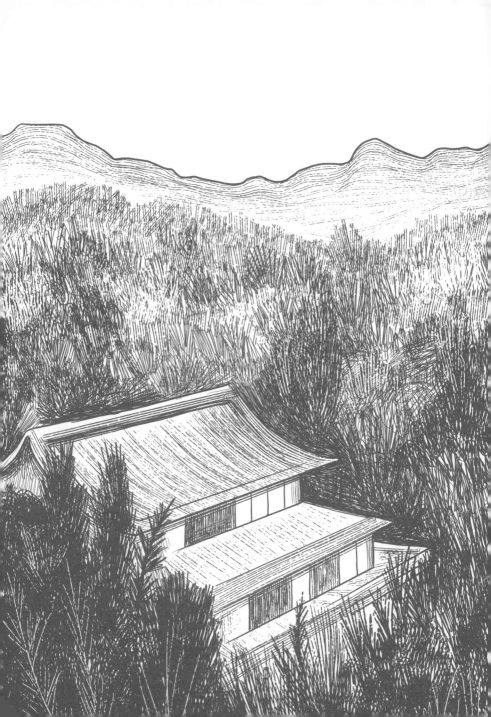

Switch Off with Self-reiki

Quantum physicists have discovered what reiki (pronounced *ray-key*) practitioners have known for over a century. Everything is energy. It's universal. Reiki consists of two Japanese characters: *rei*, meaning universal spirit, and *ki*, meaning vital life force.

Reiki was founded by Japanese Buddhist Mikao Usui. On his retreat on holy Mount Kurama Yama, he experienced *satori*, the Buddhist term for awakening or enlightenment. Usui used this powerful, newly acquired light to heal himself, developing Usui Reiki. It was his intention to share reiki so that everyone could benefit from this potent healing practice.

Today, reiki is used around the world to manage stress, for relaxation and to treat insomnia, anxiety and pain. Studies from the University of Pittsburgh School of Nursing indicate that reiki therapy may be an effective intervention to manage pain and anxiety in conjunction with traditional medicine.

Exercise: Reiki.

The reiki system of healing clears stagnant *ki* (energy) and can help you to rebalance. It is founded on five principles: do not be angry; let go of worry; be grateful; work honestly; be kind to all living things. A reiki practitioner usually receives an attunement from a reiki master to channel life force. Even though you may not have received an attunement, with a few simple steps you can practise your own self-healing using the principles of reiki.

1. Get into a comfortable position, sitting, standing or laying down, whatever feels good for you. Relax your body.

2. Centre yourself by focusing on your breath. Use a grounding meditation, following the breath all the way in and all the way out. Settle into a gentle breathing rhythm.

3. Set an intention for healing to take place. Reflect on the five principles of reiki as you focus on what you want to achieve.

4. Move the palms of your hands slowly and intentionally from your crown chakra down through each energy centre until you come to your root chakra.

5. Remember, the reiki energy is moving through you, not coming from you. The movement of *ki* through your palms will remove blocks of stagnant or stale energy.

6. When you've finished, offer a prayer of gratitude to the universe.

The Healing Power of Turmeric

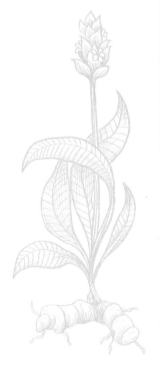

Turmeric, the bright-orange powder from the root of *Curcuma longa*, has been central to the ancient practice of Ayurveda for thousands of years. The scientific world backs up this ancient wisdom with studies confirming turmeric's ability to help manage inflammatory conditions like arthritis, reduce anxiety, aid memory, lower blood glucose and improve kidney health. More recently, studies have found that turmeric even provides the body with a feel-good hit of serotonin and dopamine. You can add it to soups, stews, curries, teas, scrambled eggs, baking, salad dressings or try a comforting turmeric latte.

Turmeric latte recipe

Caffeine free, this easy-to-make latte is the ultimate self-care bedtime beverage. You'll need one cup of milk or plant milk, a pinch of black pepper, a sweetener of your choice (date paste or maple syrup work well) and one teaspoon of freshly grated turmeric (or powder if you can't get fresh), and cinnamon or cacao to sprinkle on top.

1. Combine the ingredients and mix with a handheld blender until lump free.

2. Transfer the mixture to a saucepan and heat until hot but not boiling.

3. Pour into a mug, sprinkle with cinnamon or cacao and relax.

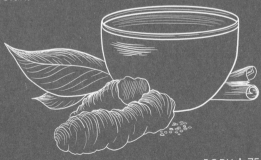

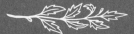

Oral Hygiene with
Oil Pulling

The ancient Indian remedy of oil pulling (*kavala-gandusha*), sometimes referred to as 'oil swishing', is a centuries-old oral hygiene practice. Used to promote healthy gums and teeth, it is growing in popularity – and with good reason. Studies suggest that this Ayurvedic remedy may reduce bacteria and plaque when used in conjunction with regular dental hygiene practices.

Ayurvedic medicine believes oil pulling to be as effective as its modern counterparts at preventing tooth decay and loss. Think of oil pulling as an ancient mouthwash pulling toxins (*ama*) from the mouth. Typically, pulling lasts five to twenty minutes and can be done with any edible oil, such as coconut, sesame, sunflower or olive oil.

Once you settle into a regular oil pulling routine, you can begin to personalize your mix, adding a few drops of essential oils. Great healing oils to include in your home oil apothecary include myrrh, clove, peppermint, spearmint, lemon, cinnamon and orange.

Exercise: Coconut oil pulling

Coconut's natural lauric acid has antibacterial and antimicrobial properties, which makes it the perfect choice for oil pulling. If you invest in a jar, remember that coconut oil also doubles as a plumping and hydrating facial cleanser. Oil pulling is usually performed first thing in the morning but can be done at any time of day.

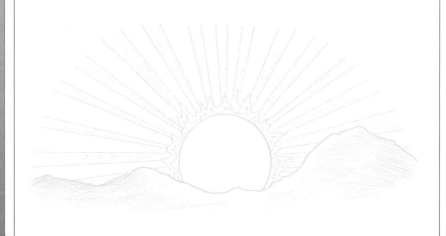

1. Take one tablespoon (or as much as you are comfortable with) of pure/virgin coconut oil.

2. Vigorously swish the oil around your mouth for as long as you are comfortable. Pull the oil through the teeth and around the mouth. Be careful not to swallow any (breathing through your nose instead of your mouth will help).

3. When you've finished, spit the oil into a bin or your food recycling compost pot (it will solidify and block your pipes if you spit it down the plug).

4. Finish by brushing your teeth and noticing how clean your mouth now feels.

Energize with Garshana

Dry skin brushing can be traced back to early Egyptian rituals. Found in many traditions, this beneficial massage known in Ayurvedic medicine as *garshana* (pronounced *gar-shun-nah*, meaning 'polishing' in Sanskrit) is a powerful detoxifier. Working with the lymphatic system, it aids blood flow, acts as an exfoliator and stimulates liver detoxification.

Combine your garshana with a post-brushing *abhyanga*, a warm, aromatic oil massage, for a sensory treat. Incorporate energizing essential oils from your ancient apothecary to stimulate your mind and body. The invigorating power of this therapy lends itself to early-morning routines. It's a ritual to wake you up, physically and mentally.

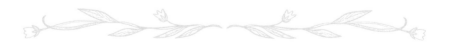

Garshana technique

You'll need a body brush with natural fibre bristles.

1. Work from your feet on dry skin with sweeping motions, applying medium to light pressure.

2. Massage towards your heart, moving from the feet to the ankles, calves, thighs, buttocks and abdomen.

3. Then, starting at the hands, move up the chest and arms.

4. Go gently on delicate areas. You're aiming for a gentle glow; it shouldn't feel uncomfortable.

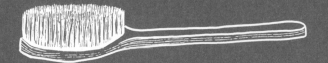

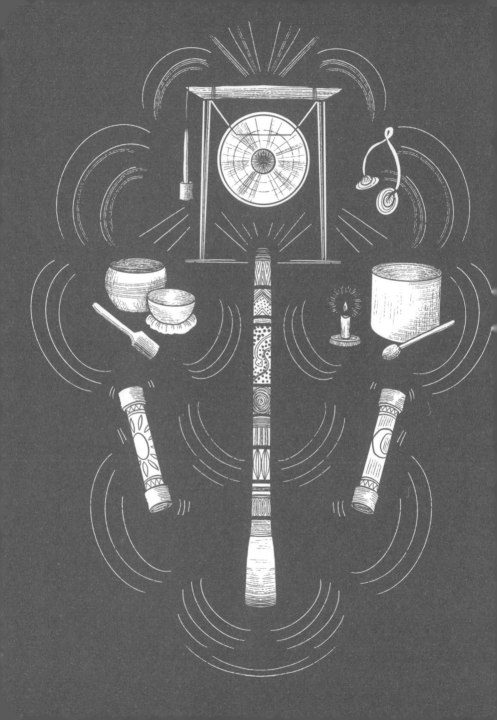

Access Inner Healing with Sound Baths

From Himalayan bowls, drums and rattles to the 40,000-year-old Australian Aboriginal didgeridoo, sound is deeply curative. Sound bathing incorporates the meditative vibrations and frequencies of gongs, bells, rain sticks, crystal bowls and singing bowls to produce a state of wellbeing. Measured in hertz, these frequencies are believed to elicit theta brainwaves, resulting in a relaxing, meditative state.

Researchers examining the effects of sound meditation found that participants reported feeling less tired, noticing a reduction in anger, tension and low mood. Moreover, they experienced an increase in spiritual wellbeing after sound bathing. The therapeutic frequencies of these ancient tools slow down our neural activity, activating the parasympathetic nervous system and allowing the body to come back into balance, away from the all too familiar fight-or-flight mode.

Exercise: Natural sound bathing

Sound bathing can be a soothing way to connect with the sounds of the natural world. Examples of organically occurring sound baths include ocean waves breaking against the shore, a gentle wind rustling the forest canopy, the tapping of raindrops against a windowpane, early-morning birdsong and the swirling of a fast-running stream over rocks.

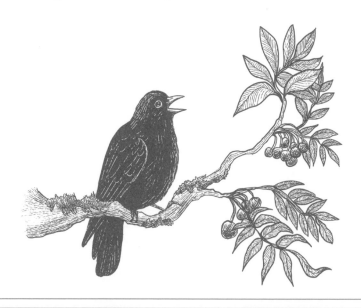

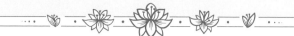

1. Find a comforting natural space where you won't be disturbed and listen. Close your eyes.

2. When you find quiet stillness in yourself, ask what you need in this moment.

3. Remain open to the sounds that present themselves. Tune into Mother Nature for an impromptu organic sound bath.

4. Set an intention. Open your eyes when you're ready.

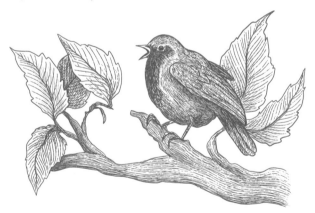

Mottainai

Mottainai translates as 'What a waste!' This ancient Japanese principle eschews throwaway culture. It's a sustainable way of thinking and living that encapsulates mindful consumption. Mottainai preserves the health of our body, our mind and our environment. It ensures that natural resources are recycled, re-used and respected.

Kintsugi, or 'golden joinery', the practice of repairing damaged ceramics with gold, is one element of mottainai. These gilded pieces are not seen as imperfect – instead they are a valued art form. It's a philosophy that we can embrace in every aspect of our lives. Kintsugi can guide our lifestyle choices, from what we purchase to how we recycle. It can help us to reflect when we encounter difficult life challenges and to see the potential for growth and a new landscape for our emotional wellbeing.

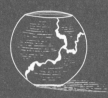

‐•°○ The mottainai challenge ○°•‐

Find ways you can prevent waste. Are there household items that you could switch to that are eco-friendly?

✦

Do you have possessions to which you are able to apply the re-use, repurpose principles of kintsugi, instead of discarding them?

✦

When you experience life's challenges, what can you take from them? How can you develop emotional kintsugi, learning from the experience to grow, emerging stronger and more resilient?

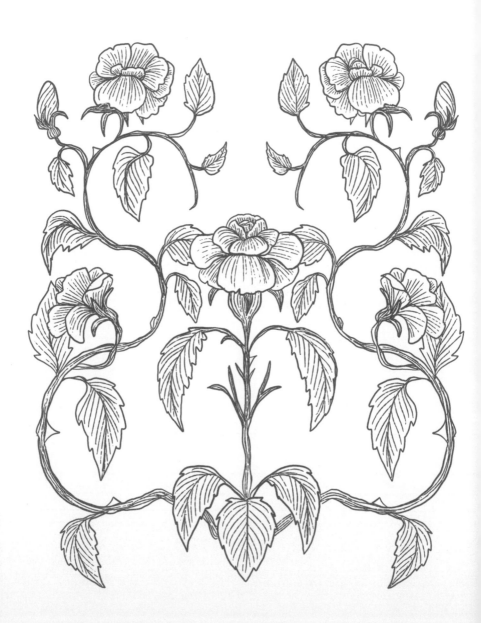

Self-care with the Sacred Rose

Roses have resonated with the human heart in art and poetry across cultures for centuries. Their velvety blooms are used in sacred rituals as a symbol of love, representing mysticism and a commitment to walking a spiritual path. For the Persian poets, the rose was a powerful muse, signifying divine love. The goddesses Aphrodite and Venus are depicted wearing them in classical mythology. The rose is a floriferous cradle of inspiration for artists and storytellers around the world.

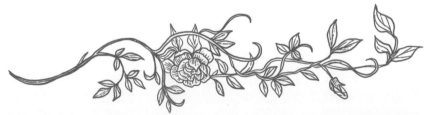

Rose beauty balm recipe

Rose oil is naturally anti-inflammatory and bursting with antioxidants to calm, moisturize and protect the skin's barrier. What's more, the fatty linoleic acid in rose oil provides hydration, revitalizing and plumping the skin. You can use this beauty balm as a hand cream, nourishing mask or body balm. Store in a cool, dry place, where it will keep for up to a year.

You'll need:
100g (⅔ cup) shea butter
50g (⅓ cup) rosehip oil
50g (⅓ cup) jojoba oil
50g (⅓ cup) beeswax
20g (¼ cup) dried rose petals
Five drops of rose oil
Five drops of lavender oil
Five drops geranium oil
A pan, a heatproof bowl, clean jars

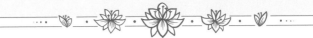

1. Fill a medium-sized pan with water. Place a heatproof bowl in the pan so that it sits securely. Warm gently.

2. Add all the ingredients to the bowl except the essential oils. Stir until melted.

3. Take the pan off the heat and remove the bowl. Take out the rose petals and discard. Allow the balm to cool for three to four minutes.

4. Add the essential oils to the mix and whisk until blended. Pour into glass containers. Label and date your jars.

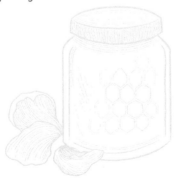

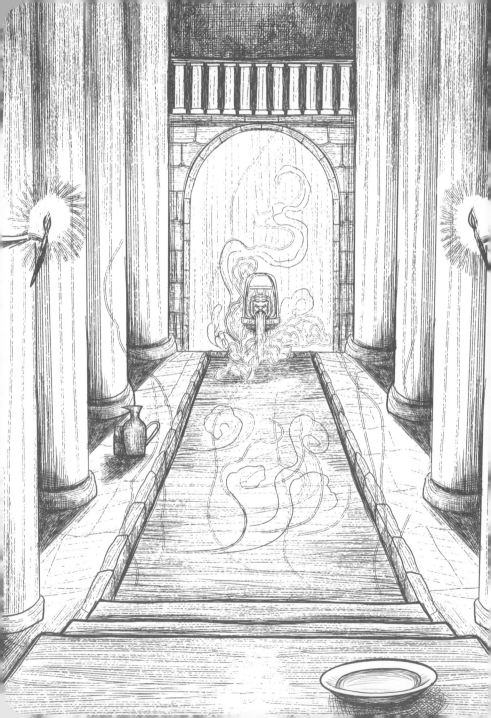

Relax with Medicinal Bath Rituals

Through the ages, tales have been spun of queens and empresses creating elaborate bathing rituals. While modern-day historians believe it's doubtful that Cleopatra bathed in a legendary concoction of milk and honey, we do know that the lactic acid found in milk has long been used to slough away dead skins cells. What the Egyptians couldn't have known, but modern science now recognizes, is that beta hydroxy acids (BHA) in milk leave the skin feeling smooth, soft and radiant.

From European spa towns to Greek bathhouses, bathing rituals have endured since civilization began. When a long day leaves you overwhelmed, a restorative soak is a sublime way to cleanse your body and mind. Embrace and revive your inner goddess by incorporating these ancient rituals into your bathing routine.

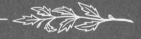

Bathing rituals

Create a relaxing environment with low lighting and candles. Compose a playlist of relaxing music and choose from the essential oils below to create your desired ritual.

✦

Energize: Used in Asia for a rejuvenating, energy-cleansing bath, coffee grounds will leave your skin feeling radiant. Add a cup to your bath or mix with coconut oil as an exfoliating scrub to use in the shower.

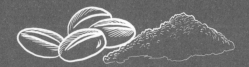

De-stress: Add a few drops of neroli oil to combat stress and anxiety.

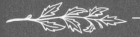

Sleep: A natural cleanser, citrusy bergamot has properties that have been found to reduce blood pressure, making it a useful component of your pre-bedtime sleep hygiene routine. Pair it with lavender to amplify its therapeutic benefits.

Focus: Zesty lemon, basil, peppermint, pine or rosemary will get you in the zone.

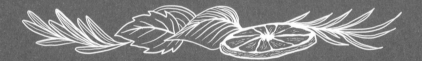

Glow: Bathing in green tea is believed to be anti-inflammatory, enhancing the complexion. Pour yourself a cup and then place a couple of green tea bags into your tub for a sustaining soak.

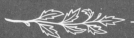

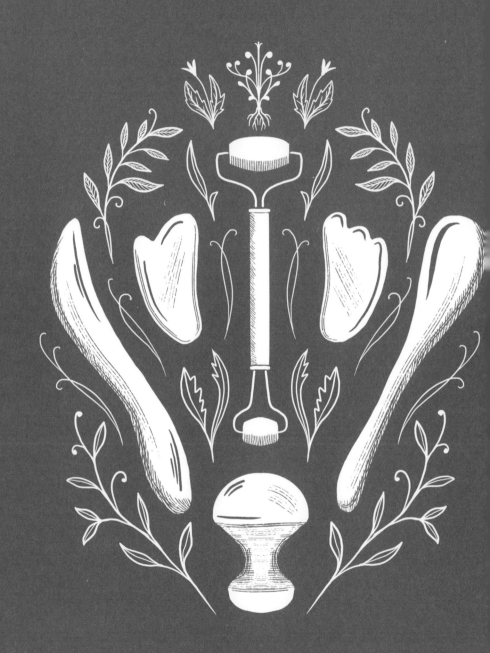

A Healing Massage with Gua Sha

The traditional Chinese medicine practice of *gua sha* has been relied upon as a healing remedy for hundreds of years. Also known as cao gio and spooning, this therapy can be traced all the way back to the Palaeolithic Age. Traditionally, stones were used to massage the body from head to toe for the management of illness and chronic pain.

Gua sha has been catapulted into modern-day usage as a deeply relaxing facial massage. It is an absorbing and meditative self-care practice. It helps us to press pause on a stressful, preoccupied yang lifestyle through creating yin, slowing our frenetic pace and activating our parasympathetic nervous system. The flow of yin and yang is restored as we learn to step in balance with our *qi*, or life-force energy. This relaxing ritual can be effortlessly incorporated into your self-care routine and will help to improve circulation, reducing puffiness and inflammation of the skin.

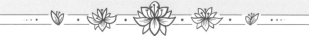

Gua sha daily ritual

You can do this first thing in the morning or last thing at night. If you're using it to de-puff, place your tool in the fridge for thirty minutes before you begin for a beautifully cooling effect. Three times a week, for ten minutes each time, is the recommended frequency for lasting results.

1. Wash and dry your hands before you begin. You'll need a gua sha stone or you can use the back of a spoon.

2. Apply moisturizer, serum or facial oil over your face and neck to stop your tool from pulling the skin.

3. Holding the curved side of your tool to your face, gently sweep in downwards strokes from the chin to the collar bone to increase circulation. Work from the centre of the throat and then along each side of the neck. Sweep five times on each area.

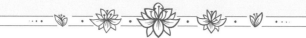

4. Moving onto the face, use outward, upward motions and light pressure. Keep your tool as close and flat to the face as possible. Slide it mindfully, going extra lightly around your eye area.

5. Continue moving over your jaw, chin, cheeks and forehead, finally flicking your stone gently up towards your hairline and over your scalp if you'd like to.

6. Wash your tool and hands in warm soapy water and notice how relaxed you feel.

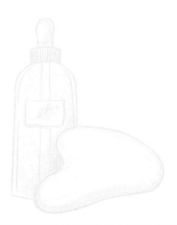

Inner and Outer Beauty with Plant-based Masks

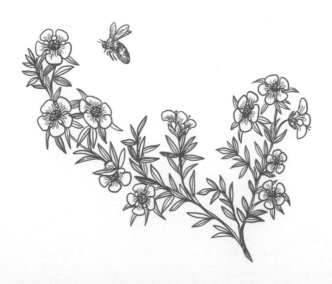

Creating your own face masks with plant-based ingredients is great for your wellness and the environment. Natural cosmetics made with love create a harmony, inside and out.

Manuka honey

Manuka honey is an anti-inflammatory, antibacterial powerhouse. Procured from the manuka bush (*Leptospermum scoparium*) in New Zealand, this healing honey is a sought-after beauty staple. Used by the indigenous Maori population, the native manuka tree provided wood and rongo (medicine) for centuries.

Today, this ancient remedy is used to treat wounds, burns, dermatitis and eczema. It's also an exceptional addition to your natural beauty store cupboard. The curative properties of this natural healer are so potent that incorporating it into any face mask will positively impact your skin.

Apply unadulterated manuka to your face and neck as a mask. Leave for fifteen minutes and remove with warm water and a soft cloth. Or you can create a homemade body scrub by mixing two tablespoons of manuka with half a cup of sugar. Use liberally in the bath or shower. You can also apply manuka topically to pimples or small cuts and grazes for accelerated healing.

Strawberry

A member of the rosaceae family, strawberries have a long history of medicinal use. The Romans believed that the roots and leaves of wild strawberries improved mood and reduced fever in the body. Chile's indigenous Mapuche people used the plant to treat indigestion and gastric complaints. Mapuche folklore told how the fragrance of ripe strawberries could fend off demons, or *weukufu*, protecting the wearer.

Packed with antioxidant vitamin C, strawberries are heart-shaped, anti-inflammatory wonders. What's more, they smell divine, creating an energizing aromatherapy all of their own. A sumptuous strawberry face mask will provide your skin with a radiant glow along with a sensory experience.

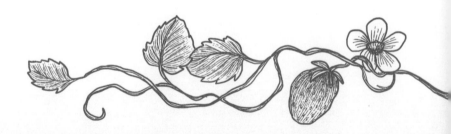

You'll need ten fresh strawberries to make a mask, along with one tablespoon of coconut or jojoba oil, one teaspoon of Manuka honey and a bowl. Using a fork or hand-held blender, mash the strawberries until smooth. Add the oil and honey, mixing into a paste. Apply to your face and leave for fifteen minutes. Rinse off with lukewarm water and pat your face dry.

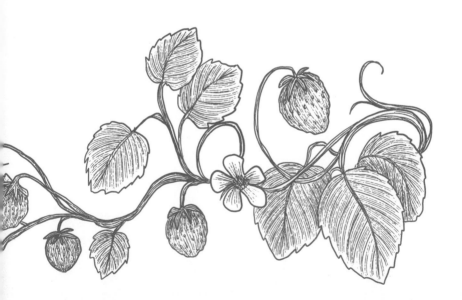

— ∘ ∘ ∘ Avocado ∘ ∘ ∘ —

Thought to be native to Puebla, Mexico, the botanical benefits of the avocado (*Persea americana*) have been prized for over 5,000 years. Named *āhuacatl* by the Aztecs, this fruit has an ancient history. Used as currency and to represent the fourteenth month of the Mayan calendar (*K'ank'in*), once upon a time avocados were even offered as a token of respect to rulers. It was believed that the avocado could also accelerate the healing of bruises, as well as providing strength and fortitude.

A natural emollient, skin-nourishing avocado is full of essential fatty acids that will hydrate and smooth your skin. The flesh of this potent superfruit is packed with collagen-boosting vitamin C and E, which will clarify your skin and leave it feeling balanced and moisturized.

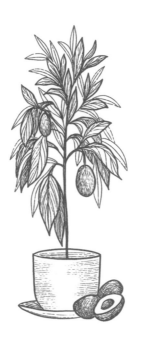

You'll need half an avocado, a teaspoon of Manuka honey, two drops of lavender oil and one teaspoon of water. Mash the avocado and mix in the other ingredients to form a smooth paste. Apply to the face and leave for fifteen minutes. Rinse off with tepid water and gently dry your face.

Spirit

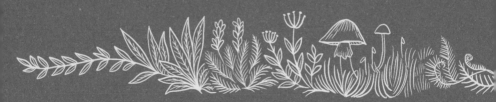

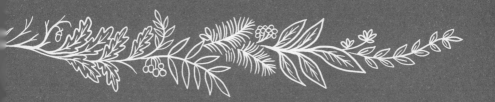

Spirituality is an often-ignored aspect of wellness. Many of us feel a disconnection; the sense that something is missing. Our spirit is inextricably linked to our mind and body. We cannot separate or compartmentalize the three; they form a wellness trinity. Spirituality is our internal compass. 'Spirit' is your journey into ancient wisdom traditions, offering a roadmap to reconnect with the sacred. This is soul medicine. These centuries-old tools and practices facilitate a deep sense of spiritual and emotional healing.

Whether it's cleansing heavy energy with a limpia ceremony or opening your heart with Mama Cacao, these earth-honouring practices will help you to elevate your consciousness. In this section, the invitation is to step into your personal power, intentionally connecting with your soul's purpose.

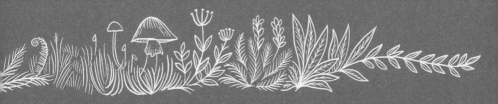

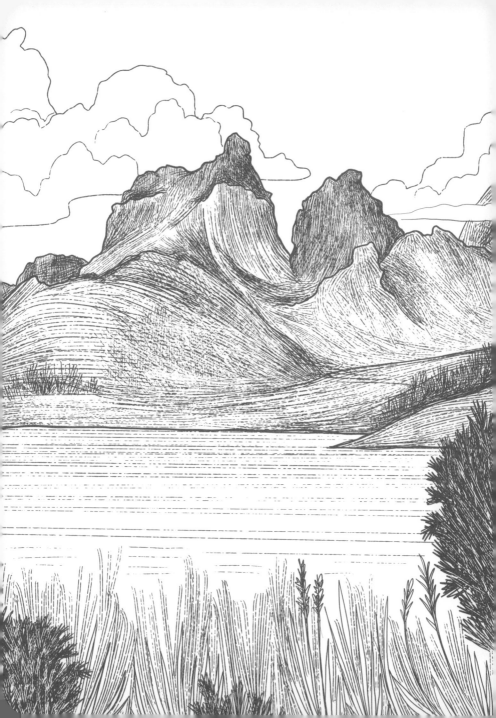

Restore Equilibrium with Limpia

We encounter a multitude of energies each day – at work, during difficult conversations, when commuting, socializing with family and friends, or through unplanned interactions. That's a huge amount of energy that we're constantly connecting with and it can create a residue. At times, being around some people in charged situations leaves us feeling heavy and depleted.

Limpia is Spanish for 'to cleanse'. A tradition stretching as far back as the Aztecs, this ritual is used to purify and cleanse the spiritual energy field of any disharmony. When you feel overwhelmed by external energies, a limpia ceremony will restore your equilibrium. Traditionally conducted by medicine women and men, you can perform your own version of a traditional limpia with the following simple ceremony.

Limpia ceremony

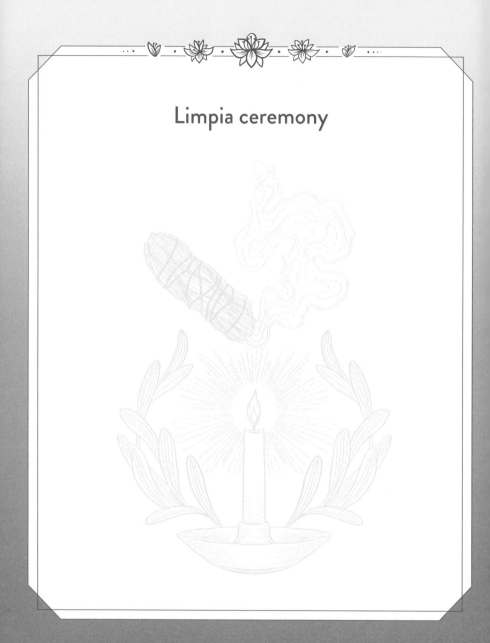

1. Create a bundle of fresh aromatic herbs and twigs.

2. Tie the herbs together and pass the bundle over your body. Sweep the herbs in front of you, behind you, under your arms and feet, and over your head to absorb any heavy energy.

3. When you've completed your sweeping, take the bundle, place it on the ground and stamp on it to release the heavy energy.

4. Replace the old energy that you've cleansed with something else, such as a homemade cleansing mist, using a tincture from your ancient apothecary.

5. Once you've finished, hold a candle in your hands. Send a prayer to the universe that this symbolic candle will bring harmony and light into your life.

Open Your Heart with a Cacao Ceremony

Indigenous cacao keepers believe that each plant has a spirit. Drinking cacao produces a higher state of awareness and understanding. When you're in this elevated state of consciousness, you can connect directly with the cacao spirit, releasing the wisdom of this sacred plant.

Packed with phytochemicals, cacoa is a prebiotic powerhouse containing antioxidants, iron, magnesium, calcium and polyphenols. It encourages the release of dopamine and serotonin, key players in human happiness and optimism. Research suggests that cacao may also reduce stress, improve blood flow to the brain, act as a natural antidepressant and lower blood pressure.

To preserve the integrity of the ceremony, whenever you are working with plant medicine like cacao, preparation and care is necessary. It must also be 100 per cent pure cacao, with nothing added. That means that your regular hot chocolate powder won't do the job. Much of the world's cocoa is harvested by indigenous communities. When you're working with ancient traditions, it's important to support Fairtrade stockists that buy directly from the farmers, recognizing and respecting the indigenous communities from whom these rituals have come.

Cacao ceremony

You'll need two tablespoons of chopped or grated ceremonial cacao and enough hot water or plant milk (dairy is believed to interfere with the absorption of flavonoids) to fill a cup. Add a natural sweetener to taste, such as honey, maple syrup or date paste (refined sugar should not be used in a ceremony). You can add cardamom, cinnamon, turmeric, nutmeg, vanilla, orange zest or chilli to flavour. Mix the ingredients together with a whisk until smooth.

1. Prepare your ceremonial cacao in advance and choose a cup for the ceremony.

2. Prepare yourself by centering with meditation or breathwork.

3. Open wiracocha and create a sacred space (see pages 39–41).

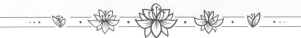

4. Set an intention for your ceremony. What will you call in? Wellness? Resilience? Love? If you'd like to manifest something, visualize it.

5. Pour the cacao into a cup. Consciously connect with the spirit of this healing plant and express gratitude.

6. Inhale the aroma of the cacao. Notice the colour, texture and sheen.

7. Sip the cacao slowly and deliberately. Mindfully come into the present moment and notice how it feels in your mouth. Consider the flavour and consistency.

8. Pay attention to your thoughts and feelings. Notice unfolding wisdom or guidance to realign with your soul's purpose.

9. Finish the ceremony by expressing gratitude, and close your sacred space.

The Healing
Power of Trees

Trees are essential to the concept of wellness. Guardians of the forest with a collective intelligence, trees are an integral part of the ecosystem. They supply oxygen, habitat, food, shade and shelter. Trees appear in folklore and mythology throughout history, and many are revered as sacred. In the ancient world of the Celts, Greeks, Vikings, Druids and beyond, trees were believed to possess metaphysical properties. The Greeks believed that trees inhabited by nymphs could foretell prophecies and connect the human world with a mystical reality.

Tree planting has long been performed as a symbolic ritual to celebrate love, marriage, birth and death. Wishing or *clootie* trees can be found at many sacred sites with brightly coloured ribbons adorning their branches. The ancient Celts worshipped trees as guardians to the otherworld, believing their roots provided a connection to the unseen realm of the ancestors. More recently, scientists have begun to investigate the healing power of trees.

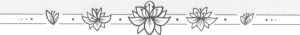

Celtic tree meditation

Research suggests that being in the presence of trees is good for our mental health. One study in Japan found that fifteen minutes spent walking in a forest decreased anxiety, confusion, fatigue and hostility. Another study discovered that living near trees lowers the stress hormone cortisol and affects our brain structure, which means we're better able to manage stress. Trees can teach us to be more mindful, strengthening our relationship to the natural world.

1. Find a tree in your local landscape. Bring your awareness to your breath. Breathe. You don't need to *do* anything. Simply bring an attitude of kindness to your meditation: whatever happens, notice it without judging.

2. As you focus on each in breath and out breath, open up to a connection with the tree.

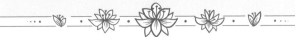

3. See if it's possible to deeply connect with the energy and spirit of the tree. Notice if the tree has a message for you, wisdom to share or a story to tell.

4. If you feel called to, tie a ribbon or *clootie* to the tree with a prayer. Offer blessings, love and gratitude to the tree.

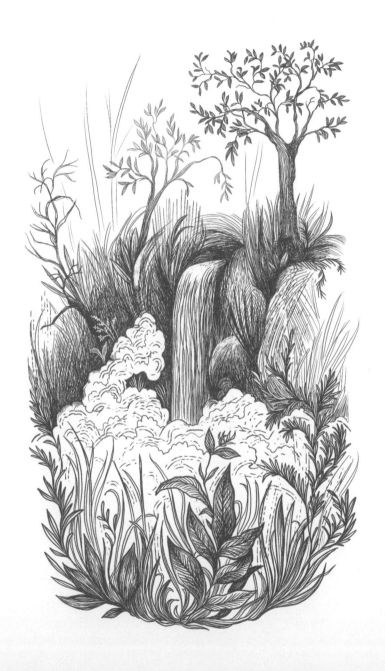

Healing and Cleansing Waters

Ancient Hindu, Buddhist, Shamanic and Tao spiritual traditions honour the life-giving energy of water with ceremony. Water is acknowledged as the essence of life and revered in many faiths and cultures with the universal archetype of the water goddess. Around the world, sacred water ceremonies are used for healing, purification and honouring the earth.

You can work with this ancient practice to give thanks, set intentions, call positive energy into your life and let go of what no longer serves you. Performing a water ceremony to express thankfulness incorporates the healing practice of gratitude, as well as reconnecting us with the natural world.

Simple water rituals

Ritual washing is practised around the globe in many religious traditions, including Christianity, Islam, Judaism and Hinduism. Using the purifying properties of water, we can integrate these principles to cleanse our energy field of heavy energy. On those days when you've been around mood-hoovers or are feeling drained, these water cleansing practices will revive and renew your wellness.

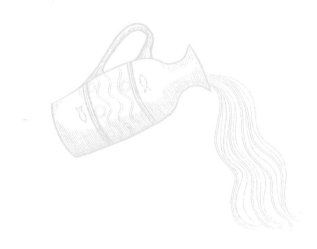

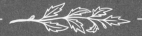

1. Salt has been used around the globe for centuries to spiritually cleanse heavy and stagnant energy. Taking an epsom (magnesium) salt bath is still practised today to purify your energy field, banishing the day's emotional rubble. Lift your mood by adding a cup of salts to your bath or soaking your feet in a bowl of salt water. You could also add a few drops of your favourite oil to soothe your aura.

2. Place your hands under running water, visualizing the transmutation of heavy energy as the water cleanses, giving that energy back to Mother Earth as it drains away.

3. Create a cleansing ritual by standing under a shower after a difficult day, allowing the water to wash away stress and anxiety.

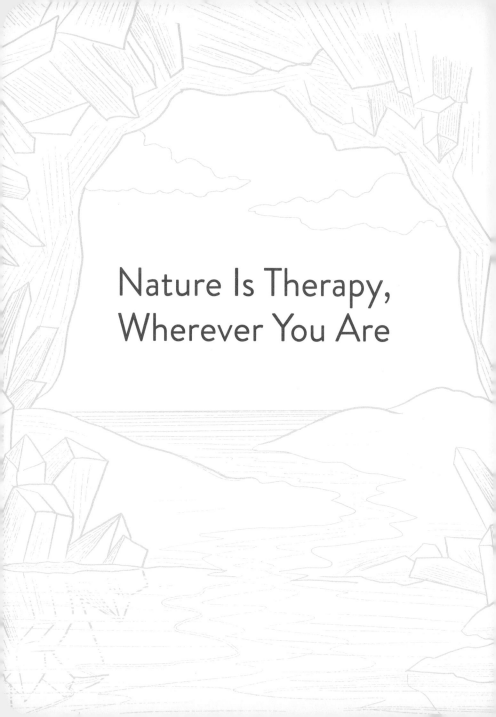

Nature Is Therapy, Wherever You Are

The power of place is recognized in many sacred natural sites around the world. Whether it's the golden beauty of Australia's sandstone Uluru, the towering peak of Mount Kailash, the purifying waters of the Ganges or the UK's Glastonbury Tor and neolithic henges, sacred sites have held spiritual significance around the globe for millennia. You may have your own natural sites near you that are considered sacred spiritual places – rivers, lakes, mountains, forests, springs, trees, hills, lagoons or caves.

We can learn to find the sacred in our own local landscape, connecting with it to recharge, renew and promote serenity. These magical locations are our personal power places, restoring our internal balance. They mark the fundamental relationship between the human spirit and the ecosystem in which we exist. This is an ethos that you can take with you wherever you go on the pale blue dot that we call home. Listen to the whisper and discover your personal sacred place.

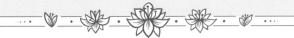

Discovering your personal power place

Collective power places like Stonehenge in the UK may be on the tourist map, but your unique power place may only be known to you. You can have more than one and it doesn't need Google maps, a signpost or fanfare to have meaning. It's possible to learn to tune in to the energy of a location wherever you are to find a personal power place. Earth-honouring traditions have used the following steps:

1. Consciously tune in to your local landscape. Where do you feel drawn to? Be open to guidance from the universe.

2. Connect with the energy. Where do you see clearly and feel connected? Which sites leave you feeling deeply attuned to the flow of life minus the overwhelm? Does self-healing feel enhanced here? These are all signs of a power place.

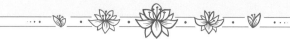

3. Are there areas where you feel dissonance? A palpable resistance to going there? The places with heavy, oppressive energy or absence of light don't have the right vibrational frequency to be your power place.

4. Identify a potential power place and set an intention to explore it.

5. Find a place to sit and create *kangaeru supēsu* (space for reflection). Contemplate.

6. When you're ready to leave, in animistic cultures it's customary to create an offering of thanks. This could be a mandala, a 'thank you' or gratitude blown into a leaf.

About the author

Gill Thackray is a writer and performance psychologist. She helps organizations and individuals globally to create conscious transformation and positive change. She has lived and worked with indigenous communities around the world, in Southeast Asia and China, studying the science of healing and ancient wisdom traditions. Gill is currently a PhD candidate researching indigenous healing practices and eco-psychology. You can find out more about her work at www.gillthackray.com

About the artist

Anna Stead is a self-taught illustrator who works from her home in the beautiful North Cotswolds, in the heart of England. She is inspired by nature, mythology, history, folklore, literature and the mythic arts, and works primarily in pen and ink. She set up Thistle Moon Studio in 2016, www.thistlemoon.co.uk, and enjoys working on a variety of custom orders and commissions. Follow her on Instagram, @thistlemoon.